NEPHRO KNOWLEDGE SERIES

Understanding Kidney Disease

Your Top 50 Questions With Simple Answers!

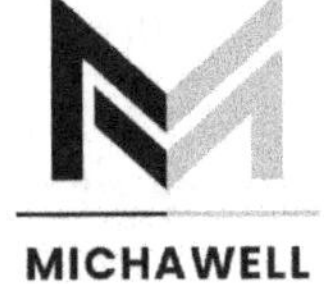

MICHAWELL

Contents

Introduction

Kidney disease is widespread both in the United States and around the world. In the United States alone, approximately 37 million people, or about 14% of adults, are estimated to have kidney disease. However, kidney disease is not a condition that is discussed much. Unless you know someone who needs kidney replacement therapy (such as dialysis or a kidney transplant) or sees a nephrologist (a kidney doctor), you might not be aware of the problems that occur when these bean-shaped organs misbehave. Your primary care provider may send you to the kidney doctor due to a lab test, and you may not even feel sick!

This book offers a simple guide to kidney disease and what you can do to keep your kidneys healthy. Please note that while this book attempts to explain the basics of kidney disease, it does not replace seeing a medical professional.

1

Understanding Kidney Disease

1. What are the kidneys?

The kidneys are organs about the size of a fist located in the back of the body (the retroperitoneal space). People typically have two kidneys, though a patient can rarely be born with only one. They can also have one functional kidney when one of the kidneys shrinks (either from lack of blood flow or poor urine drainage from the kidney).

2. What is the anatomy of the kidneys?

Each kidney has blood supplying it from the renal artery and drains via a renal vein. The kidney empties urine down a tube called the ureter into the bladder. At a microscopic level, the kidney is made of cells called nephrons. On average, a healthy human kidney contains approximately 800,000 to 1.5 million nephrons.

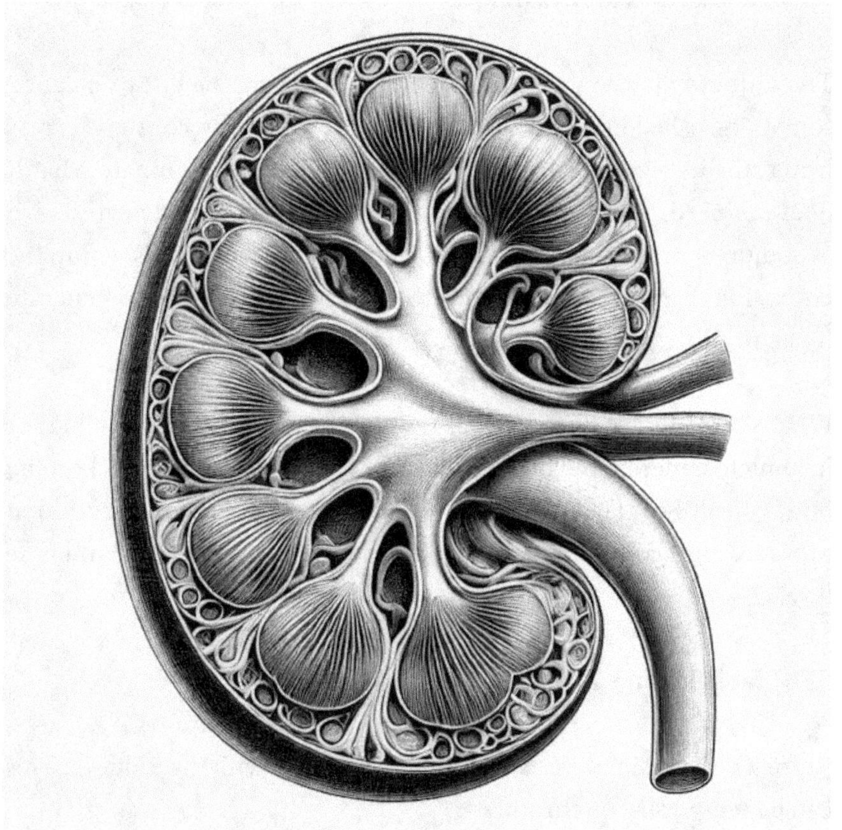

A diagram of the kidney showing the renal artery, vein, and ureter.

3. Can you live with only one kidney?

Even if you are born with one kidney or have one functioning kidney, the remaining kidney can work hard to take the place of both kidneys! This adaptability is remarkable, allowing a person to live with one kidney. In fact, it enables people to donate a kidney to another person who needs a kidney transplant and still lead a normal life!

4. What do the kidneys do?

The kidneys play an essential role in maintaining the body's balance, something called homeostasis. For instance, when you consume excess water, the kidneys retain what the body needs and eliminate what it does not need. They perform a similar function with electrolytes, such as sodium, potassium, and calcium, maintaining their levels within the body. Furthermore, throughout the body, many processes generate waste products, and the kidneys eliminate these.

What you may not know is that the kidneys are also responsible for helping to generate red blood cells and play an integral part in keeping bones healthy. They are also very important in regulating blood pressure and maintaining a balance between the body's acid and base levels.

5. What is kidney disease?

Kidney disease simply means there is a problem with the kidneys. This can be temporary or chronic.

6. What are the reasons for kidney disease?

The most common causes of kidney disease are diabetes and high blood pressure. Both conditions lead to extra stress on the kidney and, eventually, scarring. Other causes of kidney problems include inflammation of the kidney filters called glomerulonephritis, recurrent kidney infections, kidney blockages, kidney stones, autoimmune conditions, and genetic issues such as Polycystic Kidney Disease.

Temporary kidney problems typically occur when patients are sick with infections, heart problems, or dehydration.

2

Symptoms and Diagnosis

7. What are the common symptoms of kidney disease?

Early-stage kidney disease often has no symptoms. As it progresses, symptoms may be non-specific and include fatigue, swelling in the extremities, shortness of breath, nausea/ vomiting, blood in the urine, frequent urination, or high blood pressure that is difficult to control.

8. How is kidney disease diagnosed?

Kidney Disease is diagnosed based on labs and imaging. Your provider will likely talk to you about and reference a couple of labs during your visit. The first lab is called "creatinine." Creatinine is a substance made in the muscle and cleared out by the kidney. If this creatinine number is higher, the kidneys cannot clear this out appropriately. Thus, the kidneys are not working as well as they should be (although this is not always the case in patients with above or below muscle mass).

We use the creatinine and plug it into an equation to get an "eGFR" or estimated glomerular filtration rate. You can think of this as a kidney percentage. Unfortunately, as you age, the kidneys do not work as well as they used to. In fact, by the time you get to 100 years old, the kidneys may be functioning at 40 percent just by natural decline!

Your provider may also reference something called "proteinuria." Protein should not be present in excess amounts in the urine. If it is, this means there is a problem with the kidneys keeping protein in the bloodstream. Your provider may refer to a specific type of protein called "albumin."

Sometimes, there are signs of kidney problems on imaging, such as CT scans or kidney ultrasounds. There may be smaller-than-expected kidney size and evidence of scarring, kidney stones, and kidney blockages. These are used to help diagnose kidney disease.

9. My doctor told me I have "chronic kidney disease." What is this?

An individual can have a short-term or long-term problem with their kidneys. Chronic kidney disease is a kidney problem that has lasted for at least three months.

10. What are the stages of chronic kidney disease?

We stage kidney disease based on the labs and imaging described above. Please note that when eGFR is over 60, you must have another kidney problem, such as protein in the urine, kidney cysts, blood in the urine, or a kidney stone, to diagnose chronic kidney disease.

Stage	Description	Glomerular Filtration Rate (GFR)
Stage 1	Kidney damage with normal kidney function	90 or above
Stage 2	Kidney damage with mild loss of kidney function	60-89
Stage 3a	Mild to moderate loss of kidney function	45-59
Stage 3b	Moderate to severe loss of kidney function	30-44
Stage 4	Severe loss of kidney function	15-29
Stage 5	Kidney failure (end-stage renal disease)	Less than 15

11. What is acute kidney injury (AKI), and how does it differ from CKD?

You may hear a kidney problem described as acute kidney injury, sometimes called acute renal failure. This kidney problem occurs over a short period but could also become chronic kidney disease.

Common causes of acute kidney injury include dehydration, heart failure, infection, low blood pressure, kidney inflammation, kidney stones, enlarged prostate, and certain medications. Patients with CKD can also get acute worsening of their kidney disease.

12. Who do I see for kidney disease?

A physician specializing in the kidneys is called a nephrologist. An adult nephrologist first goes to medical school and then does a residency in internal medicine. Once they finish their residency, they undergo specialized training in nephrology, called a fellowship.

There are also kidney doctors for kids. These are called pediatric nephrologists, who first train in pediatrics and then specialize in pediatric nephrology.

You may see an advanced practice clinician, such as a physician assistant or nurse practitioner, who cares for patients with kidney disease.

There are also specialized nephrologists who care for patients with kidney transplants.

13. Should I see a nephrologist or urologist?

A urologist is a surgical specialty for those with kidney disease, similar to a heart surgeon to a cardiologist. They perform surgeries for kidney stones and cancers as well as procedures for kidney blockages. They also treat problems with the bladder, reproductive organs, and prostate. The urologist and nephrologist work closely together.

14. Why must I see *another specialist* when I feel fine?

Most people know that when you have chest pain, you see a heart doctor or belly pain, you see a GI doctor. However, you may not understand why you need to see a kidney doctor.

Most patients will not have symptoms at the beginning of kidney disease and may be referred to the kidney doctor due to lab abnormalities alone. It is essential to follow the recommendations of your primary care provider if they feel you need to be seen by a specialist, even if you do not feel sick.

3

Risk Factors

15. Who is at risk for kidney disease?

There are a couple of higher-risk groups for kidney disease.

- *Diabetes* is the leading cause of kidney disease, as high blood sugar can cause damage to the kidneys over time.
- Patients with *hypertension* (high blood pressure) are also at increased risk for kidney disease, as hypertension can damage the blood vessels in the kidneys.

Furthermore, patients with a family history of kidney disease have increased risk, as does older age (risk increases over 60 years old), obesity, heart disease, smoking, and certain chronic medications.

Lastly, certain ethnic groups, such as African Americans, Native Americans, Asian Americans, and Hispanic Americans, have a higher risk of kidney disease compared to the general population.

4

Prevention and Lifestyle Changes

16. How can I prevent kidney disease?

While kidney disease cannot always be prevented, managing the above risk factors and making lifestyle changes is critical to lowering the risk of kidney disease.

Important interventions include:

- Managing diabetes and blood pressure
- Eating a healthy diet
- Staying hydrated
- Avoiding smoking
- Exercising regularly
- Limiting alcohol
- Maintaining adequate weight
- Controlling high cholesterol
- Seeing your primary care provider regularly

17. What dietary changes can help protect my kidneys?

Overall, healthy eating is important for your kidneys and the body as a whole. Eating a diet rich in fruits, vegetables, whole grains, and lean proteins is essential. You should limit sugar, salt, and unhealthy fats.

18. How important is hydration for kidney health?

Hydration is essential for kidney health! Proper hydration helps the kidneys function more efficiently. Hydration is critical for waste removal, prevention of kidney stones, blood pressure regulation, electrolyte balance, and urinary tract health. However, sometimes, with more advanced kidney disease or in patients with heart problems, your provider may discuss limiting your fluids.

19. What role does exercise play in kidney health?

Exercise plays a significant role in maintaining kidney health and preventing kidney disease. Regular physical activity helps manage risk factors associated with kidney disease. Exercise improves blood pressure control, helps with your blood sugars, aids in weight loss, enhances cardiovascular health, and improves inflammation.

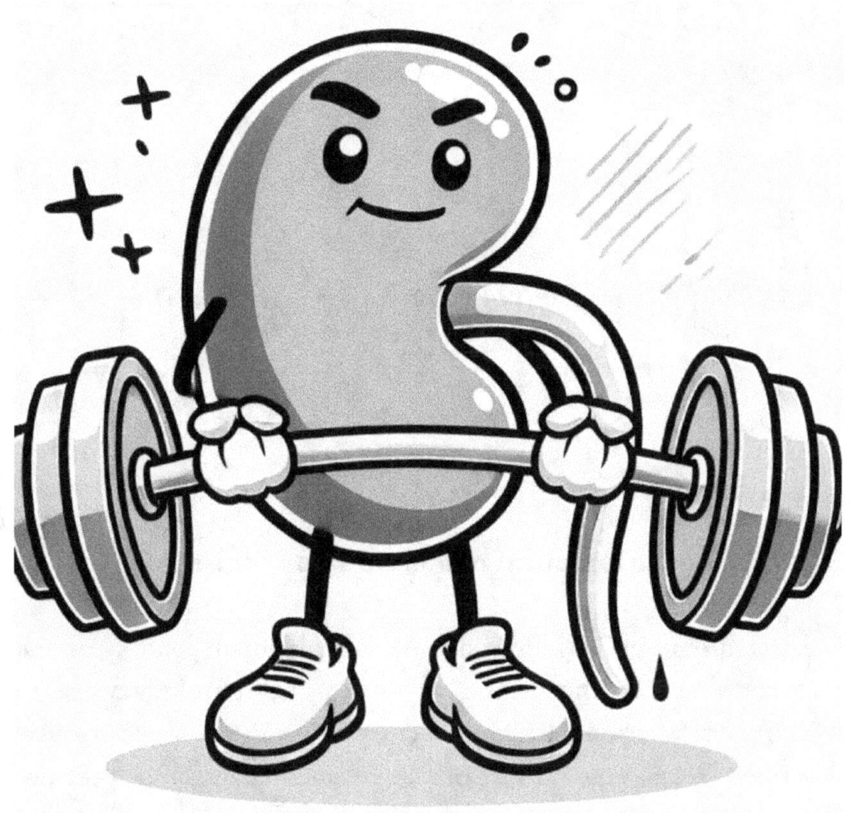

5

Treatments and Management

20. What are the treatment options for kidney disease?

Treatment options for kidney disease vary greatly depending on the stage and severity of the disease. Early stages of chronic kidney disease (CKD) often focus on managing underlying conditions as previously described. Regular monitoring of kidney function and blood pressure is crucial.

Treatment may involve medications to manage symptoms and complications in more advanced stages, such as low blood counts and bone disease.

When kidney function declines significantly, treatments like dialysis or a kidney transplant become necessary to replace the lost kidney function.

21. What medications are commonly prescribed for kidney disease?

Medications commonly prescribed for kidney disease aim to control symptoms, manage complications, and overall work to slow the progression of the disease. These include antihypertensive drugs to control high blood pressure, such as ACE inhibitors and ARBs, which help protect kidney function.

Diuretics may be prescribed to reduce fluid retention and swelling. Phosphate binders are used to manage high phosphorus levels in the blood. Erythropoiesis-stimulating agents (ESAs) help treat anemia by stimulating red blood cell production.

Additionally, medications to control blood sugar levels in diabetic patients, such as insulin or oral antidiabetic drugs, are essential for protecting kidney health. Your provider may also discuss using newer diabetes medications for CKD (called SLGT2 inhibitors, even if you do not have diabetes).

Sometimes, the reason for your kidney disease is an inflammatory process. You may be on medications to suppress your immune system in that case.

22. What medications should I avoid with chronic kidney disease?

- Over the counter pain medications, including, but not limited to, Ibuprofen, Naproxen, and Diclofenac, are called non-steroidal anti-inflammatories or NSAIDs. These can hurt the kidneys over time and should be avoided unless absolutely needed.
- Medications for constipation, such as magnesium-containing laxatives or phosphate-containing enemas, should be avoided.
- Proton pump inhibitors, used for indigestion, can increase the risk for chronic kidney disease, and an alternative medication should

be considered if possible.
- It is also recommended to limit iodinated contrast if the benefits are less than the kidney risks.
- Lastly, it is recommended that you check with your provider before starting any over-the-counter supplements.

23. What is end-stage renal disease (ESRD)?

End-stage renal disease (ESRD) is the final stage of chronic kidney disease, where kidney function has deteriorated to less than 15%. At this stage, kidneys can no longer effectively filter waste products, maintain fluid and electrolyte balance, or produce essential hormones.

24. What is dialysis, and when is it needed?

Dialysis is a medical procedure that performs the kidneys' functions when they can no longer work adequately. Unfortunately, dialysis does not fix the kidneys but replaces what they should otherwise be doing. Dialysis removes waste products, excess fluids, and toxins from the blood.

There are two main types of dialysis: hemodialysis and peritoneal dialysis. Hemodialysis involves cleaning the blood through a machine outside the body. Peritoneal dialysis uses the lining of the abdomen to filter blood inside the body.

Dialysis is a critical intervention to maintain life and manage the symptoms and complications of kidney failure.

25. How does a kidney transplant work?

A kidney transplant involves surgically placing a healthy kidney from a donor into a person with end-stage renal disease. The new kidney takes over the work of filtering blood, allowing the patient to live without dialysis.

There are two types of kidney transplants: living-donor transplants, where a kidney is donated by a living person (often a family member or friend), and deceased-donor transplants, where the kidney comes from a recently deceased donor.

The recipient's immune system must be carefully managed with medications to prevent rejection of the new kidney. A successful kidney transplant can significantly improve the quality of life and longevity for people with severe kidney disease!

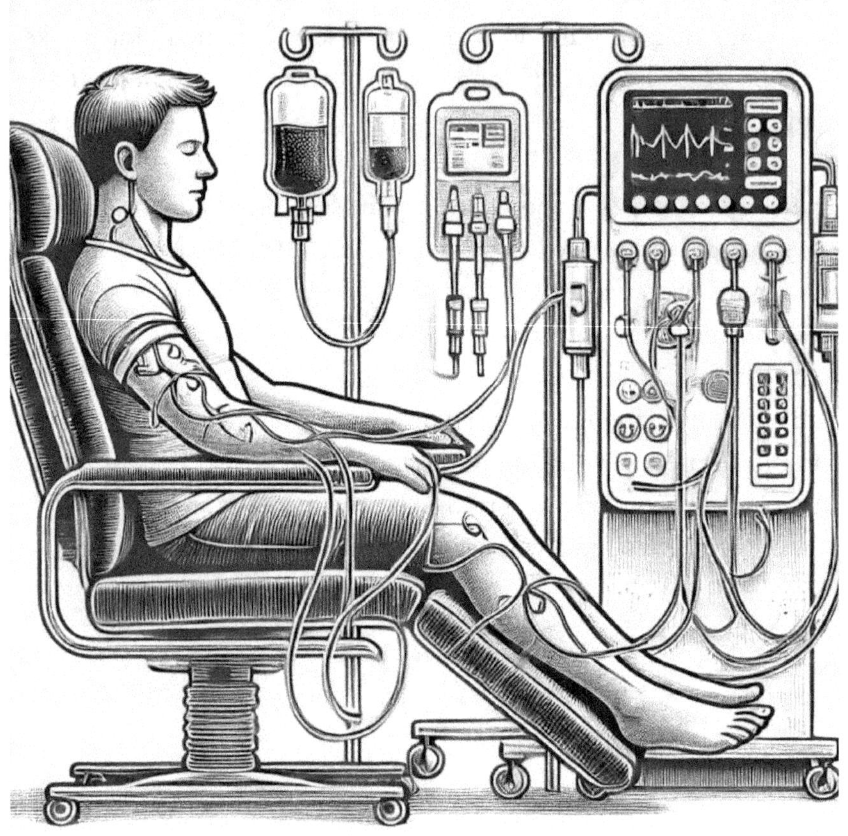

6

Living with Kidney Disease

26. How can I manage kidney disease on a daily basis?

Managing kidney disease on a daily basis involves a combination of lifestyle changes, adherence to medications, and regular monitoring. Regular physical activity helps maintain overall health, and it's important to manage underlying conditions such as diabetes and high blood pressure.

Taking prescribed medications as directed and keeping regular appointments with healthcare providers is essential for monitoring kidney function and adjusting treatment as needed. Tracking your health metrics, such as blood pressure, weight, and blood sugar levels, can help you stay on top of your condition.

27. What dietary restrictions should I follow?

Your provider may make specific recommendations to limit certain foods. This does not apply to every patient. Dietary restrictions for kidney disease patients may include limiting sodium, potassium, protein, and phosphorus intake. High-sodium foods, such as fast foods, should be avoided to help control blood pressure and fluid retention.

Foods high in potassium, like bananas, oranges, and potatoes, should be limited to prevent hyperkalemia (high potassium).

Phosphorus-rich foods like dairy products, nuts, and colas should also be restricted to avoid bone and cardiovascular problems.

Additionally, protein intake may need to be moderated based on the kidney disease stage and a healthcare provider's dietary recommendations. Working with a dietitian is crucial to creating a meal plan that meets your needs.

28. How can I cope with the emotional impact of kidney disease?

Coping with the emotional impact of kidney disease involves seeking support from family, friends, and healthcare professionals. It's normal to experience a range of emotions, including anxiety, depression, and frustration. Talking to a mental health professional, such as a therapist or counselor, can help you navigate these feelings.

Joining a support group in person or online can provide a sense of community and understanding from others facing similar challenges. Stress-relief techniques can also be beneficial.

Staying informed about your condition and treatment options can empower you and reduce feelings of helplessness.

29. What support resources are available for kidney disease patients?

Numerous support resources are available for kidney disease patients, including organizations like the National Kidney Foundation and the American Kidney Fund, which provide educational materials, support networks, and financial assistance.

Many hospitals and clinics offer support groups and counseling services for patients and their families. Online communities and forums can also provide valuable peer support and information.

Social workers can also help connect you with resources for managing treatment costs, transportation to medical appointments, and navigating insurance issues.

Using these resources to improve your quality of life and manage your condition effectively is essential.

30. What are the complications of advanced kidney disease?

Advanced kidney disease can lead to numerous complications, significantly affecting overall health. These complications include fluid retention, high blood pressure, and pulmonary edema.

Electrolyte imbalances, such as hyperkalemia (high potassium levels), can cause dangerous heart rhythms.

Anemia is common due to reduced erythropoietin production, leading to fatigue and weakness.

Bone disease and mineral disorders occur because of imbalances in calcium and phosphorus.

Patients also face a higher risk of cardiovascular diseases, infections due to a weakened immune system, and peripheral neuropathy.

Managing these complications often requires comprehensive care and regular monitoring by healthcare providers.

31. How does kidney disease affect other parts of the body?

Kidney disease impacts various body parts because it maintains overall homeostasis. Impaired kidney function can lead to cardiovascular issues such as hypertension, heart disease, and stroke due to fluid and electrolyte imbalances.

Bone health is compromised as kidneys fail to regulate calcium and phosphorus, leading to bone density loss and fractures. The nervous system can be affected, causing confusion, difficulty concentrating, and peripheral neuropathy. Skin issues like itching and discoloration are also common.

Additionally, kidney disease can lead to anemia, which reduces oxygen delivery to tissues, exacerbating fatigue and overall weakness.

32. What are the options for palliative care in kidney disease?

Palliative care in kidney disease focuses on relieving symptoms, improving quality of life, and supporting patients and their families. This care approach includes pain management, treating symptoms such as nausea, fatigue, and itching, and addressing emotional and psychological needs.

Palliative care teams work alongside nephrologists to provide comprehensive care that aligns with the patient's values and goals. In advanced stages, patients may opt for conservative management, focusing on comfort rather than aggressive treatments like dialysis. Palliative care also includes advanced care planning, ensuring patients' wishes are respected at the end of life.

7

Special Populations

33. How does kidney disease affect children?

Kidney disease in children can significantly impact growth, development, and overall health. Children with chronic kidney disease may experience delayed growth and development due to hormonal imbalances and nutritional deficiencies. They are also at risk for bone disease, anemia, and cardiovascular issues.

Managing kidney disease in children involves a multidisciplinary approach, including pediatric nephrologists, dietitians, and social workers, to address the unique needs of young patients. Early detection and treatment are crucial to mitigate the long-term effects and improve the child's quality of life.

34. What should pregnant women with kidney disease know?

Pregnant women with kidney disease face unique challenges and risks, including hypertension, pre-eclampsia, and preterm birth. These women must receive specialized care from nephrologists and obstetricians to manage their condition throughout pregnancy.

Monitoring kidney function, blood pressure, and electrolyte levels is essential. Medications may need to be adjusted to ensure they are safe for the mother and the developing baby. Proper nutritional support and frequent prenatal visits help manage the condition and provide the best possible outcomes for both mother and child.

35. How does kidney disease impact the elderly?

Kidney disease disproportionately affects the elderly, who are already at higher risk due to age-related decline in kidney function. In older adults, kidney disease can exacerbate existing health issues such as hypertension, diabetes, and cardiovascular diseases. The elderly may also experience more pronounced symptoms and complications, including anemia, bone disorders, and electrolyte imbalances.

Management often requires a careful balance of medications, diet, and lifestyle changes to accommodate other co-existing conditions. When planning treatment strategies, it's essential to consider the overall health and functional status of elderly patients.

36. What are the considerations for kidney disease in minority populations?

Minority populations, including African Americans, Hispanics, Native Americans, and Asians, face higher rates of kidney disease due to genetic, socioeconomic, and healthcare access factors. These groups are also more likely to have conditions such as diabetes and hypertension, which are significant risk factors for kidney disease.

Addressing kidney disease in minority populations involves:
- Improving access to healthcare.
- Increasing awareness and education about kidney disease.
- Addressing social determinants of health.

Culturally competent care and targeted public health initiatives are crucial to reducing disparities and improving these communities' outcomes.

8

Research and Future Directions

37. What are the latest advancements in kidney disease research?

Recent advancements in kidney disease research include the development of new biomarkers for early detection and improved diagnostic techniques. Research also focuses on regenerative medicine and stem cell therapies to repair damaged kidney tissue. Advances in genetics and genomics are helping to understand the hereditary aspects of kidney disease, leading to personalized medicine approaches.

Additionally, novel drug therapies are being developed to target specific pathways involved in kidney disease progression. Innovative technologies, such as wearable devices for continuous monitoring of kidney function, are also emerging.

38. How can I participate in kidney disease research?

Patients can participate in kidney disease research by enrolling in clinical trials, which test new treatments and therapies. You can find clinical trials through databases like ClinicalTrials.gov or by contacting major medical centers and research institutions.

Patient advocacy groups and organizations like the American Society of Nephrology and the National Kidney Foundation often provide information about ongoing research studies. Participants may provide biological samples, complete surveys, or test new medications under medical supervision.

Discuss with your healthcare provider to understand the benefits and risks before participating.

39. What is the future outlook for kidney disease treatments?

The outlook for kidney disease treatments is promising, with ongoing research focusing on innovative therapies and better management strategies. Advances in gene editing, such as CRISPR, can correct genetic defects causing kidney disease. Regenerative medicine and bioengineering aim to develop artificial kidneys and repair damaged tissues. Improved dialysis techniques and less invasive options are being explored.

Additionally, personalized medicine promises tailored treatments based on individual genetic profiles. Continued investment in research and development is expected to lead to more effective and accessible treatments.

9

Miscellaneous Questions

40. Can kidney disease be reversed?

Kidney disease can sometimes be slowed or stabilized in its early stages with appropriate treatment and lifestyle changes. However, kidney disease is not generally reversible. Managing underlying conditions such as diabetes and hypertension, adhering to a kidney-friendly diet, and taking prescribed medications can help prevent further damage. In advanced stages, the focus shifts to managing symptoms and complications and preparing for treatments like dialysis or transplantation.

41. What is the role of alternative medicine in kidney disease treatment?

Alternative medicine, including dietary supplements, herbal remedies, and acupuncture, is often used to complement conventional treatments for kidney disease. However, it's essential to consult with a healthcare provider before using alternative therapies, as some may interact with prescribed medications or worsen kidney function. Evidence supporting the efficacy of alternative treatments varies, and they should not replace standard medical care.

42. How does kidney disease affect life expectancy?

Kidney disease can significantly impact life expectancy, especially in its advanced stages. Factors influencing prognosis include the stage of the disease, underlying health conditions, age, and the effectiveness of treatments. Early detection and management of risk factors can improve outcomes. Patients with end-stage renal disease (ESRD) who undergo dialysis or receive a kidney transplant can extend their life expectancy. Still, they require ongoing medical care and lifestyle adjustments.

43. What are the financial implications of kidney disease?

Kidney disease can lead to substantial financial burdens due to the costs of treatments, medications, and frequent medical appointments. Dialysis and kidney transplants are costly. Patients may face additional costs for transportation, dietary modifications, and potential loss of income due to illness. Health insurance can help cover some expenses, but out-of-pocket costs can still be significant. Financial assistance programs and patient advocacy organizations may provide support and resources to help manage these costs.

10

Resources and Support

44. Where can I find more information about kidney disease?

Information about kidney disease can be found on the websites of prominent health organizations such as the National Kidney Foundation, Mayo Clinic, and the National Institute of Diabetes and Digestive and Kidney Diseases (NIDDK). These sources provide comprehensive information on symptoms, treatments, research, and patient support.

45. What organizations support kidney disease patients?

Several organizations, including the National Kidney Foundation, American Society of Nephrology, American Kidney Fund, and Kidney Disease: Improving Global Outcomes (KDIGO), support kidney disease patients. These organizations offer educational resources, financial assistance, patient advocacy, and community support programs.

46. How can I connect with a kidney disease support group?

You can connect with kidney disease support groups through hospitals, clinics, and patient advocacy organizations. Online forums also provide platforms for connecting with others facing similar challenges. Support groups offer emotional support and practical advice.

11

Practical Advice

47. How can I talk to my doctor about kidney disease?

When discussing kidney disease with your doctor, be open and honest about your symptoms, concerns, and lifestyle! Prepare questions in advance, bring a list of your medications, and consider bringing a family member or friend for support. Discuss treatment options, potential side effects, and lifestyle changes you can make to manage your condition.

48. What questions should I ask during my nephrology appointment?

During medical appointments, ask about your diagnosis, stage of kidney disease, and treatment options. Inquire about the benefits and risks of different treatments, dietary and lifestyle recommendations, and ways to monitor your condition. Ask about symptoms to watch for, how to manage complications, and the frequency of follow-up appointments.

49. What practical tips can help me live well with kidney disease?

Living well with kidney disease involves:
- Following a kidney-friendly diet
- Staying active
- Adhering to your treatment plan

50. Anything else I can do?

You should monitor your health regularly, manage stress, and seek support from family, friends, and support groups. Finally, you should stay informed about your condition and engage in activities that bring you fulfillment!

12

Conclusion

Kidney disease is a complex condition that affects millions of people worldwide. Understanding the kidney's role and the factors that can lead to kidney disease is crucial for maintaining kidney health and preventing disease progression.

We hope this guide answers common questions about kidney disease, its causes, symptoms, diagnosis, and treatment options.

Managing kidney disease involves a combination of medical care, lifestyle changes, and proactive health monitoring. Early detection and intervention are vital to slowing the progression of the disease and improving overall quality of life. Patients should work closely with healthcare providers to develop a personalized care plan. Emotional and psychological support is also vital, as living with kidney disease can be challenging.

Ultimately, the best strategies for managing kidney disease are staying informed, adhering to treatment plans, and making healthy lifestyle choices.

13

References

American Heart Association. (n.d.). Exercise and blood pressure. Retrieved from https://www.heart.org/en/health-topics/high-blood-pressure/changes-you-can-make-to-manage-high-blood-pressure/getting-active-to-control-high-blood-pressure#:~=Exercise%20can%20help%20you%20manage%20blood%20pressure%20and%20more.&text=It%20can%20also%20help%20you,good%20for%20your%20blood%20pressure

American Heart Association. (n.d.). Heart disease and chronic kidney disease. Retrieved from https://www.ahajournals.org/doi/10.1161/CIRCULATIONAHA.120.050686

American Heart Association. (n.d.). Protein and your health. Retrieved from https://www.heart.org/en/healthy-living/healthy-eating/eat-smart/nutrition-basics/protein-and-heart-health

American Kidney Fund. (n.d.). Acute kidney injury. Retrieved from https://www.kidneyfund.org/all-about-kidneys/other-kidney-proble ms/acute-kidney-injury-aki

American Kidney Fund. (n.d.). Kidney disease. Retrieved from https://www.kidneyfund.org/professionals-and-research/online-c ontinuing-education

American Kidney Fund. (n.d.). Kidney disease prevention. Retrieved from https://www.kidneyfund.org/all-about-kidneys/kidney-disease-prevention

American Kidney Fund. (n.d.). Starting dialysis without a plan. Retrieved from https://www.kidneyfund.org/kidney-disease-unkn own-cause/starting-dialysis-without-treatment-plan

American Kidney Fund. (n.d.). Your kidney-friendly food: Managing phosphorus. Retrieved from https://www.kidneyfund.org/article/you r-kidney-friendly-food-plan-managing-phosphorus

American Kidney Fund. (n.d.). Potassium and your diet. Retrieved from https://www.kidneyfund.org/hyperkalemia-guidelines?utm_source= Google&utm_medium=CPC&utm_campaign=beyondbananas&gad_s ource=1&gclid=CjwKCAjwp4m0BhBAEiwAsdc4aJRmIdOWbVBrrQo WTa3esXeK_or0wye0UA5MOb_tjbKaToT-ZrlTOBoClQUQAvD_B wE

Centers for Disease Control and Prevention. (n.d.). Chronic kidney disease basics. Retrieved from https://www.cdc.gov/kidneydisease/ba sics.html

REFERENCES

Centers for Disease Control and Prevention. (n.d.). Chronic kidney disease surveillance system. Retrieved from https://nccd.cdc.gov/ckd/

Centers for Disease Control and Prevention. (n.d.). Diabetes and exercise. Retrieved from https://www.cdc.gov/diabetes/managing/physical-activity.html

Cleveland Clinic. (n.d.). Acute kidney injury (AKI). Retrieved from https://my.clevelandclinic.org/health/diseases/17689-kidney-failure

Cleveland Clinic. (n.d.). Hyperkalemia. Retrieved from https://my.clevelandclinic.org/health/diseases/15184-hyperkalemia-high-blood-potassium

Cleveland Clinic. (n.d.). Best and worst sources of protein. Retrieved from https://health.clevelandclinic.org/best-and-worst-sources-of-protein

Harvard T.H. Chan School of Public Health. (n.d.). Staying active. Retrieved from https://nutritionsource.hsph.harvard.edu/staying-active/

Harvard T.H. Chan School of Public Health. (n.d.). Protein. Retrieved from https://nutritionsource.hsph.harvard.edu/what-should-you-eat/protein/

Harvard T.H. Chan School of Public Health. (n.d.). The nutrition source: Phosphorus. Retrieved from https://nutritionsource.hsph.harvard.edu/phosphorus/

Harvard T.H. Chan School of Public Health. (n.d.). The nutrition source:

Potassium. Retrieved from https://nutritionsource.hsph.harvard.edu/potassium/

Johns Hopkins Medicine. (n.d.). Sleep better. Retrieved from https://www.hopkinsmedicine.org/health/wellness-and-prevention/sleep-better

Mayo Clinic. (n.d.). Acute kidney failure. Retrieved from https://www.mayoclinic.org/diseases-conditions/kidney-failure/symptoms-causes/syc-20369048

Mayo Clinic. (n.d.). Cardiovascular exercise. Retrieved from https://www.mayoclinic.org/healthy-lifestyle/fitness/in-depth/aerobic-exercise/art-20045541

Mayo Clinic. (n.d.). Chronic kidney disease. Retrieved from https://www.mayoclinic.org/diseases-conditions/chronic-kidney-disease/symptoms-causes/syc-20354521

Mayo Clinic. (n.d.). Nutrition and healthy eating. Retrieved from https://www.mayoclinic.org/healthy-lifestyle/nutrition-and-healthy-eating/expert-answers/fiber-supplements/faq-20058513

National Institute on Aging. (n.d.). Protein foods. Retrieved from https://www.nia.nih.gov/health/protein-foods

National Institute of Diabetes and Digestive and Kidney Diseases. (n.d.). High blood pressure and kidney disease. Retrieved from https://www.niddk.nih.gov/health-information/kidney-disease/high-blood-pressure

National Institute of Diabetes and Digestive and Kidney Diseases. (n.d.).

REFERENCES

Kidney disease statistics for the United States. Retrieved from https://www.niddk.nih.gov/health-information/health-statistics/kidney-disease

National Kidney Foundation. (n.d.). Kidney disease information. Retrieved from [https://www.kidney.org/Cares?gad_source=1&

National Kidney Foundation. (n.d.). Kidney disease treatment. Retrieved from https://www.kidney.org/atoz/content/patient-education-brochures

National Kidney Foundation. (n.d.). Living with kidney disease. Retrieved from https://www.kidney.org/category/living-kidneydisease

National Kidney Foundation. (n.d.). Nutrition and chronic kidney disease. Retrieved from https://www.kidney.org/atoz/content/nutrikidfail_stage1-4

National Kidney Foundation. (2021). Obesity and kidney disease. Retrieved from https://www.kidney.org/sites/default/files/obesity_and_ckd_workshop_agenda_20210401.pdf

National Kidney Foundation. (n.d.). Smoking and your health. Retrieved from https://www.kidney.org/atoz/content/smoking#:~=Smoking%20can%20affect%20medicines%20used,can%20make%20kidney%20disease%20worse

National Kidney Foundation. (n.d.). Weight management and kidney disease. Retrieved from https://www.kidney.org/atoz/content/obesity

National Institutes of Health. (2014). Dietary protein and muscle mass. Retrieved from https://www.ncbi.nlm.nih.gov/pmc/articles/PMC401 8953/

U.S. Department of Agriculture. (n.d.). Protein foods. Retrieved from https://ask.usda.gov/s/article/What-foods-are-in-the-Protein-Foods-Group

www.ingramcontent.com/pod-product-compliance
Lightning Source LLC
Chambersburg PA
CBHW051713250726
48653CB00007B/3006